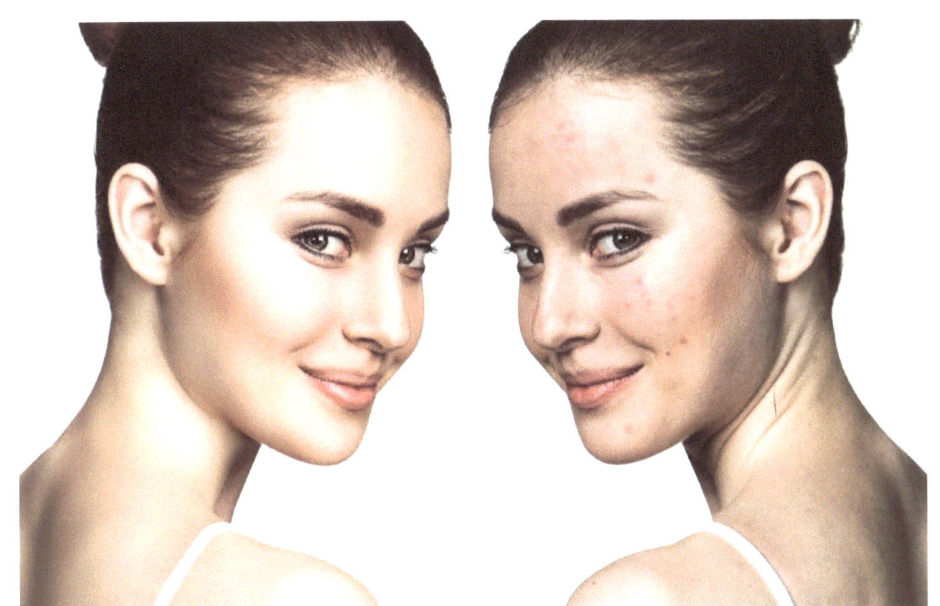

Everyday Acne Care

Introduction

This book contains information written by a United States board-certified dermatologist and is meant to assist you in care of your acne-prone skin at home. It should not replace a proper diagnosis, evaluation, and prescriptions with a dermatologist.

The word "doctor" means "teacher" in Latin, and so it is a doctor's duty to teach. I was inspired to write this book and other books in my Everyday skin care series so that I may teach others what I have taught my patients. As a teacher of skin science, I take care to be aware of the latest skin science research, and to sift through the myths and controversies. I hope that this book teaches you something.

I do not wish to promote any single brand product in this book, but I will try to give generic ingredients that are beneficial to the skin and your acne treatment when I can. To find brands that contain the recommended ingredients, you may go to www.skincreamguide.com, and search the skin product ingredient.

Chapters

CHAPTER 1: Why Do I Have Acne?

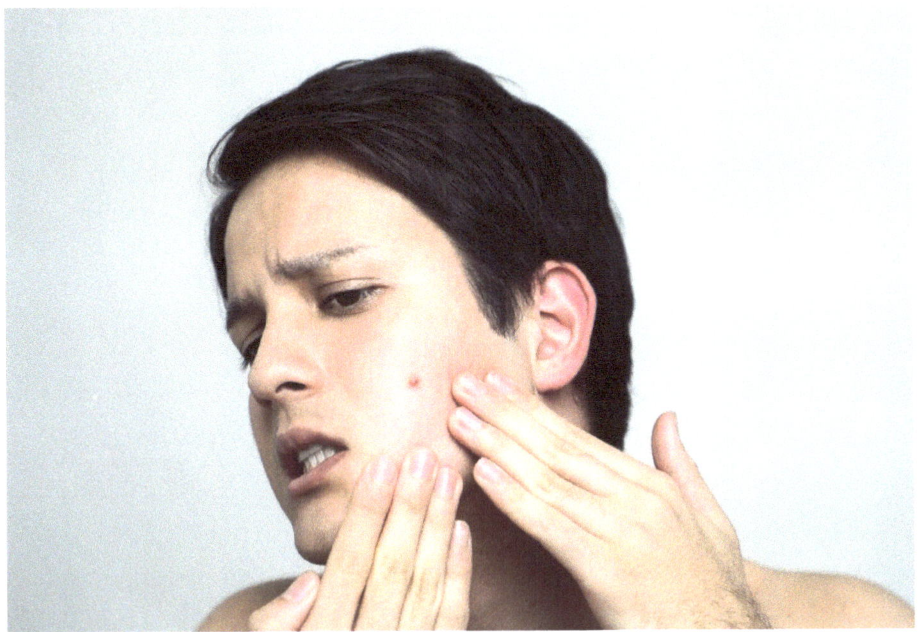

It is only natural to question why, no matter what the health problem. Dermatologists have studied acne for many years and we continue to study it and try our best to understand the cause and solution. To this day, we understand acne to be a complex process where a few necessary elements come together. I like to call these "acne elements."

The "acne elements" that create acne are as follows: decreased or inadequate monthly turnover of skin cells, excess oil (sebum) production in the skin, certain bacteria and sometimes yeast, and inflammation. The strength of each of these "acne-creating elements" may determine where on your skin your acne will appear and what type of acne. I like to think of these "acne-creating elements" as being further influenced by genetics and the environment.

Each element may be worsened by hereditary, genetic or environmental factors. For example, it may run in the family to have more androgen hormone receptors on your face. Androgens stimulate sebum production at the cellular level in our skin. Remember, sebum is one of the key acne-causing elements.

Women with polycystic ovarian syndrome have more circulating androgens. See Chapter 9 for environmental triggers (sun, food, and more) to avoid when you have acne. There are other diseases that may cause an androgen hormone surge and give acne. If you have symptoms or signs of elevated androgen hormones, it is important that you seek further evaluation and testing from your primary care physician and possibly with a specialist such as an endocrinologist.   The symptoms and signs of excess androgen hormones in women are as follows: male-pattern hair growth, frontotemporal hair loss, clitoromegaly, irregular menses, infertility, abrupt onset of severe acne, Cushing's disease features, acne that is severe or resistant to therapy, acanthosis nigricans (velvety brown plaques in skin folds), and obesity.

I wish to discuss further each "acne-creating element" so you can see why each is important and why dermatologists treat acne the way we do. Let's begin with discussing decreased skin cell turnover and what that means. Our live skin cells rise from deep epidermis to the surface until they die and flake off about every 30 days. It is believed that in acne this skin cell turnover is not working well where the dead skin cells remain stuck or caught in a pore creating a clogged pore.

We do not fully understand if that poor cell turnover is simply because of lots of oil (sebum) collecting and acting like mortar to clog the cells in the pore. We do believe that you also need the other "acne-creating elements." To address the poor skin cell turnover element, many dermatologists will advise gently exfoliating the skin. It is crucial that exfoliation is done gently or you may increase the inflammation, which is another "acne-creating element."

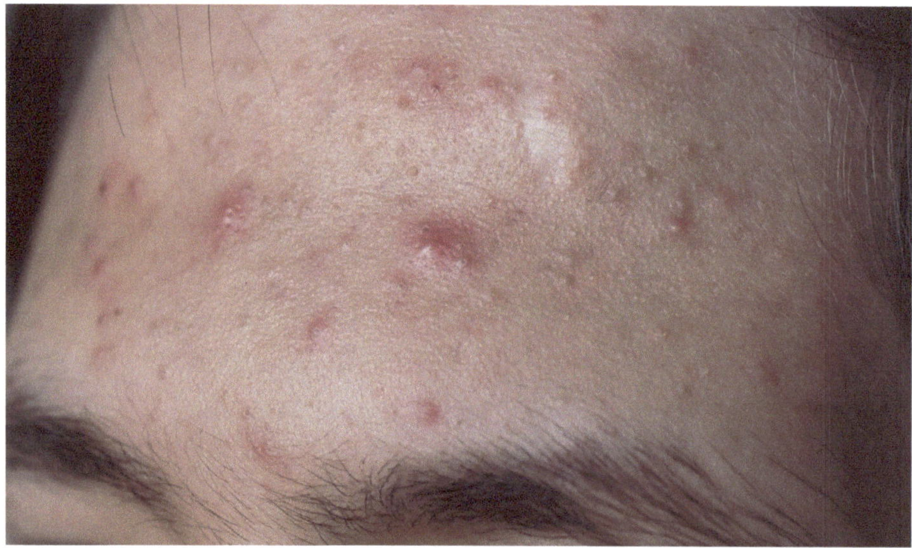

Moving on to the next "acne-creating element," we have oil (sebum) production. It seems to be increased in acne-prone skin. Oil production in the skin is linked to hormones, hereditary and sometimes environment. Some people genetically are heavier oil producers. Some people may have an excess of androgen hormones like with polycystic ovarian syndrome, or intake of oral steroids. People with poor hygiene or inadequate cleansing of their skin may allow the oil to accumulate and they may worsen their acne. This is one reason dermatologists recommend twice daily face cleansing for facial acne.

Oil and Yeast Acne

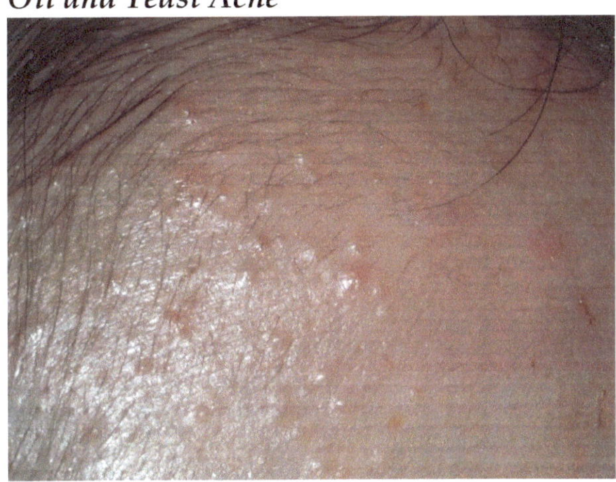

Photo courtesy of Jamanetwork.com

Buildup of skin oil (sebum) encourages yeast overgrowth on the skin. The malassezia or pityrosporum yeast normally lives on our skin as part of our normal skin flora and in harmony balanced with bacteria and even mites, but the yeast thrives in oily skin. This yeast has been associated with dandruff of the scalp and face (seborrheic dermatitis) and even acne.

In my office, I like to take a Wood's lamp (black light) and shine it on my patient's "acne", and if I can see the coral pink fluorescence of the malassezia yeast then I can confirm its presence and/or abundance and likely cause of that acne. The proof of the yeast etiology of this type of acne is that the pink fluorescence will fade or disappear where the acne fades. If you do not have a light and you suspect that you may have this yeast, then you may be able to tell yeast acne from typical acne in that yeast acne tends to be smaller/finer pink bumps, and yeast acne clusters where the oil glands are the most active: scalp, forehead, nose, medial cheeks, mid chin, mid upper chest, shoulders, and mid upper back.

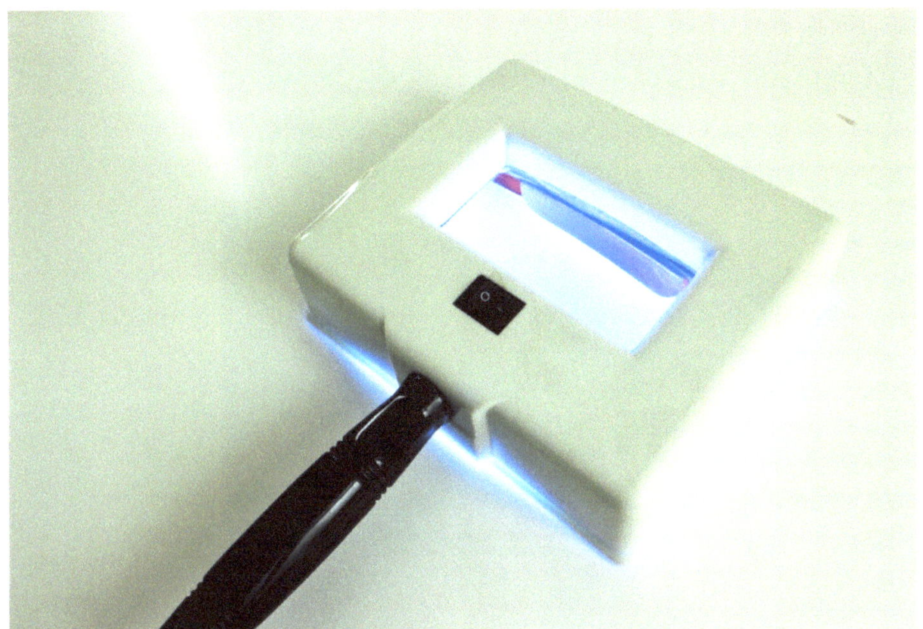

Shown above, typical Wood's Lamp used by Dermatologist

Here is the sad news about yeast acne. While it is easy to treat with topical or oral anti-yeast medications, it is often misdiagnosed as stubborn or resistant acne. I have seen many patients over the years that were told they had resistant acne requiring oral antibiotics or Accutane/isotretinoin when it cleared with a simple anti-yeast regimen. Often going on antibiotics will just make the yeast acne worse. Accutane/isotretinoin happens to work for yeast acne because it controls the oil, and the yeast is dependent on the oil, but it is like killing a fly with a hammer, and not worth the side effects when a simple, safer and brief anti-yeast regimen works just fine. Many people will have both yeast acne and typical acne, and are best diagnosed with a dermatologist. Be proactive and if you suspect yeast, ask your dermatologist to look for pityrosporum acne.

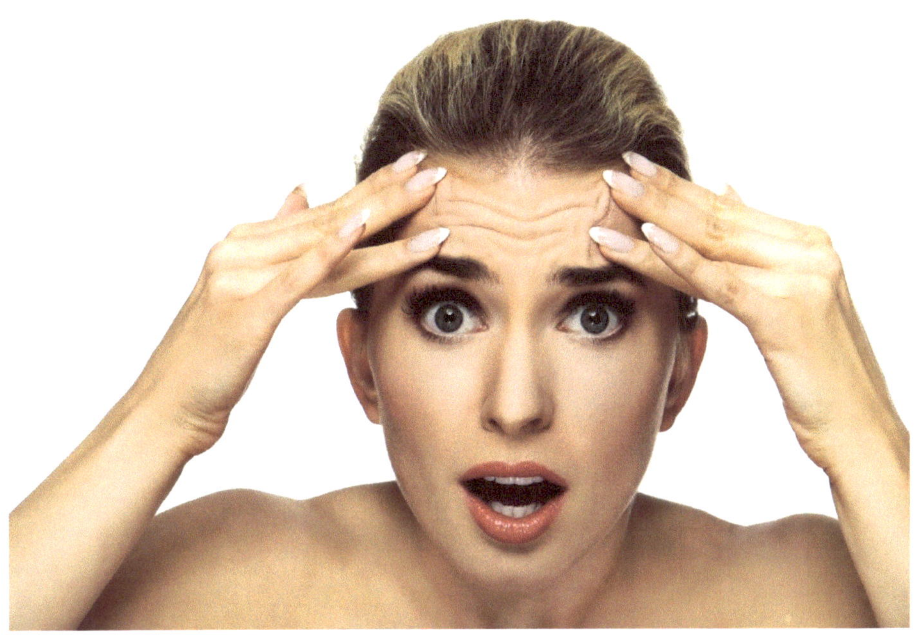

Back to our list of four "acne-creating elements" that I described at the beginning of this chapter, we are at number three: bacteria. For many years, dermatologists believed that acne was best treated with topical and oral antibiotics, and therefore acne was mostly a bacterial infection. Hopefully, you understand that this is not true, and we now understand acne to be multifactorial where bacteria is just one of the factors or "acne-creating elements" I like to call them.

Sometimes typical acne can truly get infected with bacteria, and infection predominates the problem, but that is only sometimes. It is true that scientists find "Propionibacterium acnes," a species of bacteria on the skin, associated with acne, but recent studies are finding that there are good acne-fighting and bad acne-causing versions of this bacteria. In addition, there are other studies that have yet to be completed trying to figure out whether oral probiotics and/or probiotic lotions may be helpful to fighting acne. The early studies are positive and promising, but I caution anyone who believes they can cure their acne with probiotics alone, as they are overlooking the other "acne-creating elements." Finally, antibiotics are no longer a first-line remedy for acne, and there is increased concern among doctors about bacterial resistance and other side effects of antibiotics.

Now it is time to discuss the final "acne-creating element:" inflammation. Doctors use the term inflammation to refer to redness and swelling in skin or other tissues. It is believed that acne inflammation may be triggered by bacteria, may be present with or without the bacteria, or may be from other unknown factors.   The source of inflammation in acne is currently being studied. We know more about controlling or treating the inflammation of acne, than we know about the cause. There are many natural anti-inflammatories that benefit acne but may need to be combined to approach the anti-inflammatory power of some prescription acne medications. I will discuss the treatments in later chapters.

Chapter 2: Is there a cure?

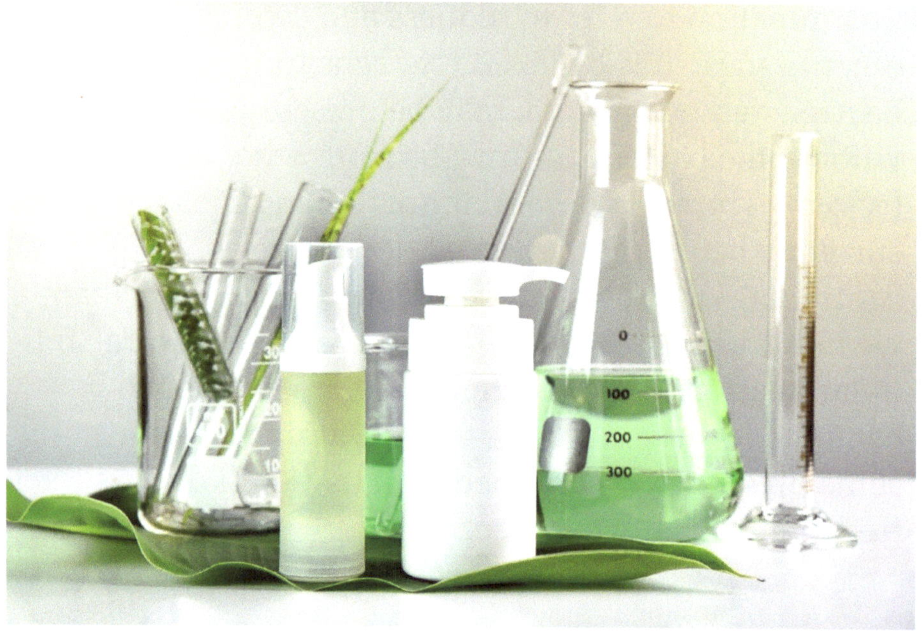

While there is hope that someday there will be a cure for acne, at this time, I am disappointed to report that there is no cure. After reading chapter 1, and learning the complicated mechanism(s) of acne, it should be no surprise that a cure would be something challenging to achieve. Many people do outgrow acne, and there are others who continue to get acne as an adult.

Even oral "Accutane", now known by the generic name of Isotretinoin, is not considered a cure by dermatologists. Many people will have one round of oral isotretinoin and seem to never have cystic scarring acne again, so it would be fair to say that isotretinoin may come close to curing cystic acne in some people. While the exact mechanism of isotretinoin is not known, it is known that it reduces the production of sebum, shrinks the sebaceous glands, and improves keratin deposition in the skin so fewer pores are clogged. Due to side effects, isotretinoin is a treatment that is usually reserved for only severe, cystic, and scarring acne. It should be discussed with careful consideration between you and your dermatologist.

While there is no cure yet for acne, it is possible to get acne under good control and prevent scarring if treatment is started promptly.

For best control of your acne, most treatments are daily and not weekly or monthly. There are some chemical peels, laser and light treatments that can help acne significantly with weekly or monthly application, but most insurance plans do not cover the cost of these treatments.

Chapter 3: A Daily Acne Fighting Routine

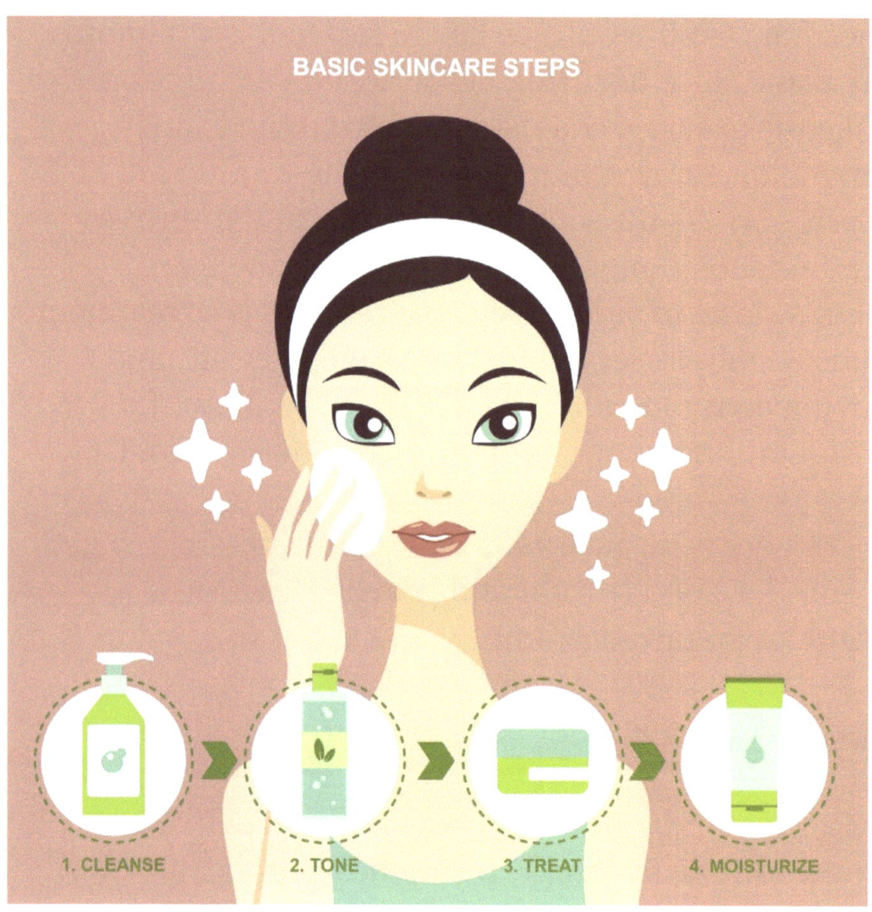

If you have acne, then you must commit to a daily routine that prevents acne as well as treats the acne. Your dermatologist may prescribe you medications to take daily, but it is not enough to use the medications. You must also avoid the triggers of acne on a daily basis. Think of it as an anti-acne lifestyle, just like if we want to stay fit and maintain our weight we must diet and exercise.

If you are reading this book to help your teenager with their acne, you are probably getting concerned after hearing that a daily routine is needed. Many teenagers have trouble following the daily routine. I recommend pairing their acne-fighting routine with other daily hygiene steps like teeth brushing or bathing, and reminding them for the first two weeks of their routine at least. The routine is more than likely going to be as follows: step 1 – cleanse, step 2 – tone, step 3 – apply medication, step 4 – moisturize or apply sunblock and/or makeup.

The following are triggers of acne or things that may make your acne worse: improper face cleansing, stress, hormone changes, over-application of occlusive moisturizers, occlusion of the skin, heredity (family genetics), high glycemic diet (sugars, carbohydrates), skim or fat free milk, certain topical oils (see Chapter 9), whey protein supplements, steroids, medications like Lithium, certain hormonal contraceptives (Mirena, Depo-Provera, Norplant). While one cannot avoid heredity, the other triggers can be controlled or avoided pretty easily.

Bottom line, with our current knowledge of the causes of acne, and current treatments, a daily commitment to a routine is necessary for best results.

Chapter Four: Cleansing and Toning for Acne

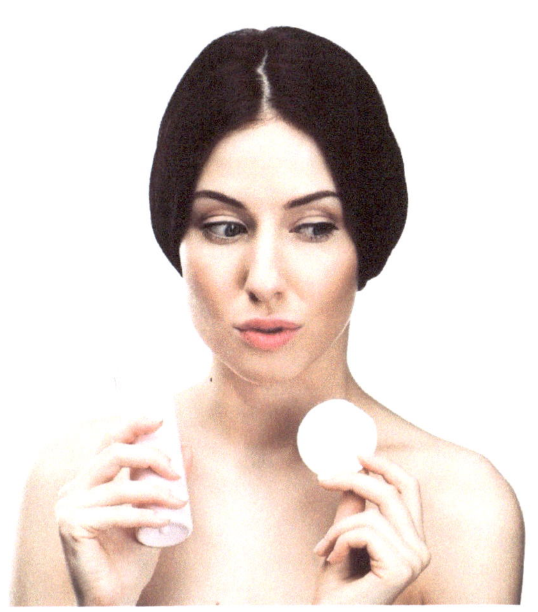

Years of studies have shown that cleansing (cleaning) your face twice a day with a mild or gentle cleanser is best to control acne. Use your fingertips, and not a washcloth or a spinning brush. Washing your face once a day or three times a day may result in more acne then if you do the recommended twice a day. If you wear makeup, then it should be a makeup that can be removed with this gentle cleansing and without extra steps or you may risk irritation.

Recent studies are showing that it is important to maintain a healthy acidic pH of our face skin to avoid acne breakouts. Before these studies, I and many other dermatologists were against toners and the toning step. The original toners on the market were more likely to irritate which can worsen acne. The best toners for acne and other inflammatory skin problems correct the skin ph. Look for a toner that corrects pH gently.   There are new and effective skin toners that balance the skin pH using Apple Cider vinegar.

I am currently against spinning brushes for acne, until there are further controlled studies. I have seen too many patients in my office try the spinning brushes and have worse or no better acne. I worry that with certain types of acne the brushes are just grinding in the oil, bacteria or yeast and not doing what the manufacturers profess. For now, I recommend gentle cleansing of the face twice a day with a mild cleanser using one's hands/fingers and no washcloth.

Chapter 5: Do I need a moisturizer?

 While acne is caused in part by excess oil (sebum) in the skin, many people who suffer from acne fear using a skin moisturizer or think they do not need one. If you use a gentle cleanser and you cleanse twice a day only as recommended, and you are a heavier face sebum (oil) producer, you are less likely to need a moisturizer or will get away with a very light moisturizer. Rather if your skin is more sensitive, you produce less sebum, and/or you experience peeling from your topical medications sometimes, then you are more likely to need a moisturizer.

If you are a teen, then you are less likely to need moisturizing than an adult. With age, we have less sebum production, and our skin is drier.
If you choose to use a moisturizer, then be sure and choose an appropriate one for your needs. The most reliable, safe moisturizers for everyone are gentle, with very few ingredients, fragrance-free, paraben-free, sunscreen-free, and dye-free. For younger people, I usually recommend a "lotion" for the face. For adults, I will recommend lotion or cream.

Many face lotions or creams nowadays contain sunscreen (SPF 15.) I recommend avoiding such moisturizers and keeping sunblock or sunscreen separate. Sunscreens carry a risk of irritating the skin. Sensitive skin or mineral sunblocks are the least irritating type of topical sun protection. They can be trusted to not aggravate or irritate your skin.

WHEN TO APPLY SUNBLOCK...
Apply the sunblock last before makeup, after cleansing, after medication, after moisturizing, but before makeup.

WHEN TO APPLY MAKEUP...
Apply makeup last, after cleansing, after medication, after lotion, after sunblock.

WHICH MOISTURIZER?

When deciding on which moisturizer is best, I prefer simple, hypoallergenic moisturizers for people with sensitive skin or if you also apply a skin medicine or serum before your moisturizer. Deciding on which moisturizer goes best with the rest of your regimen can be complicated or simple. I will begin with the simple answer.

If you are a teen, or young adult under 25, I recommend the gentle, fragrance-free, dye-free, paraben-free, hypoallergenic, sunscreen-free moisturizers. Lotion is best, if you tend to be combination or oilier skin. Cream is preferred, if you are more dry or irritated. Do not be fooled by advertisements for the latest oil or herb in the moisturizer. These additives are just not worth the risk of irritation, or allergy, as they are not standardized and subjected to clinical skin testing.

If you are an adult over 25, and you are starting to worry about signs of aging and wrinkles, then consider a moisturizer that contains antioxidants, retinols and/or (collagen/elastin stimulating) growth factors. Many of my dermatologist colleagues and I believe that retinoids and growth factors should be a lifelong skin supplement.

If you do not have sensitive skin and you wish to get the most out of your moisturizer, you may choose one that contains more power than simply moisturizing. Some moisturizers contain acne-fighting ingredients or age-fighting power or both. There are also moisturizers that help calm redness and rosacea, or fade brown discolorations and spots.

If I could simplify the task of choosing a moisturizer, I would recommend that you consider the following: 1. The degree of natural oil you collect on your face, 2. What else you are putting on your face in your daily skin treatment routine, and 3. How sensitive your skin may be. If you are still confused, most dermatologists can help you come up with a skin treatment routine that is best for your needs.

Chapter 6: Makeup and Acne

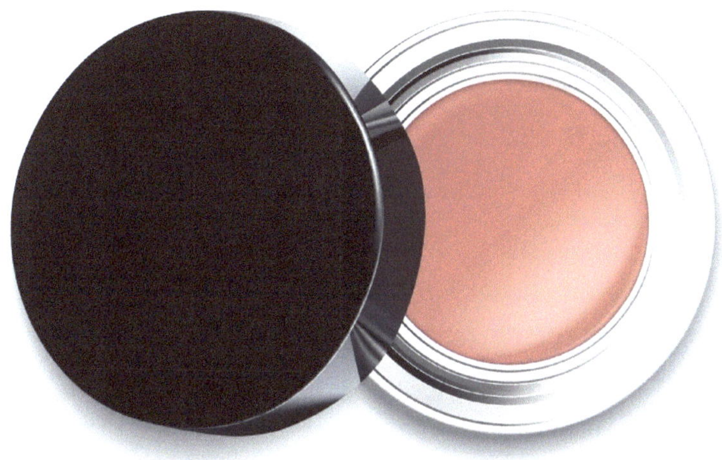

When you have acne and you wish to apply makeup, there are a few simple rules that you should follow to avoid problems or worse acne. These rules involve your choice of makeup and style of application. First, choose a makeup that is "mineral" as it will contain less chemical irritants. Second, apply makeup last: after skin medication, after moisturizer, after sunblock, after serum. See previous chapter for more about the order of things. Third, apply your makeup in thin and small quantities, so as not to further clog your pores.

Try to clean your face gently twice a day, especially if you wear makeup regularly. Do not wear your makeup to bed, as the more layers on your skin, the more to occlude your pores.   In addition, makeup can attract and collect environmental debris, pollutants, as well as microorganisms throughout the day. All of this buildup, can result in more breakouts or irritation.

Regarding technique of applying your makeup, if you have a stubborn, swollen pimple that you are struggling to cover, try an under-eye concealer. Under-eye concealers work very well to mask pimples. It should almost match or skin tone or be a shade lighter for best results. The correction pallets that contain violet, green and yellow are helpful to cover big pimples too, but require two layers where the first layer is the correction color, and the second layer is your usual makeup base color. Finish with applying a light powder to set and protect your result. Do not cake on thick layers of concealer or base as this looks unnatural and odd, and can attract negative attention.

If you would like to lightly cover up some blemishes, but you are not accustomed to wearing makeup, and need sun protection, then consider one of the tinted mineral sunblocks. They add a subtle tint of cover regardless of your skin type, and provide sunblock protection simultaneously.

Chapter 7: Sun and Acne

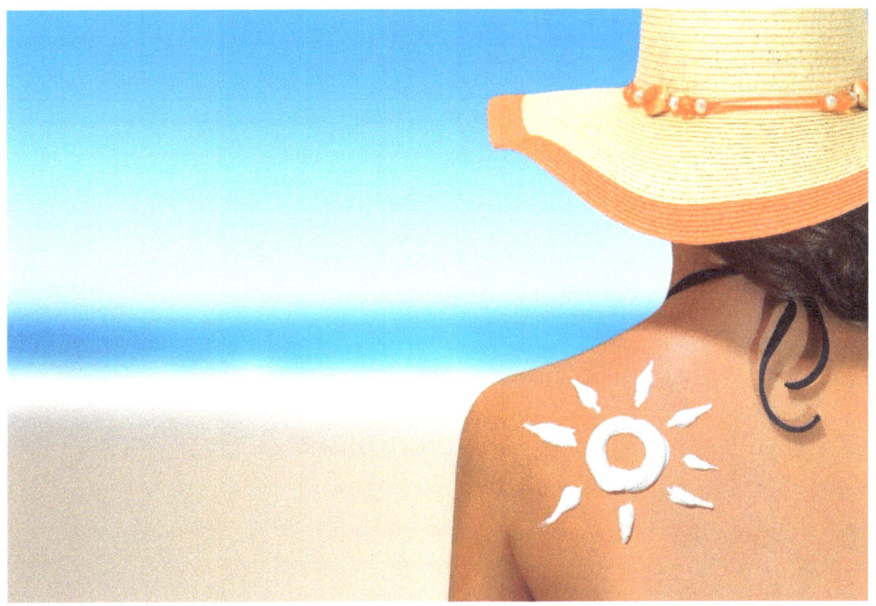

In the past, some dermatologists would advise their patients to get a little sun to calm their acne. Dermatologists do not recommend Sun exposure for acne today, because the hazards of too much ultraviolet light in sunshine outweigh any small benefit. While it is true that ultraviolet light suppresses inflammation in skin problems including acne, this benefit can be isolated and used in a safe way to treat your skin, with the new acne in-office and home low-level light devices. Unfiltered sunshine is carcinogenic or cancer causing, but we believe the low-level light is not. There are other hazards of the sun while treating your acne, beyond the carcinogenicity.

Another hazard of getting sun while treating acne, is that the sun can dry out the already dead skin cells or kill some that were not dead yet, creating a thicker dead skin cell layer. This thicker dead skin cell layer may in turn clog more pores, giving more acne. Many acne medications are sun-sensitizing as they may exfoliate the dead skin cells. This can significantly increase the risk of a sunburn or brown discoloration from the sun while treating your acne.

So hopefully you are hearing my message clearly, that sun is no good for acne-prone skin. Never go outside or sit near a window without sunblock or sun protection while treating your acne. If you are concerned about vitamin D, then you should be able to get that adequately from diet and/or supplements.

Chapter 8: Diet and Acne

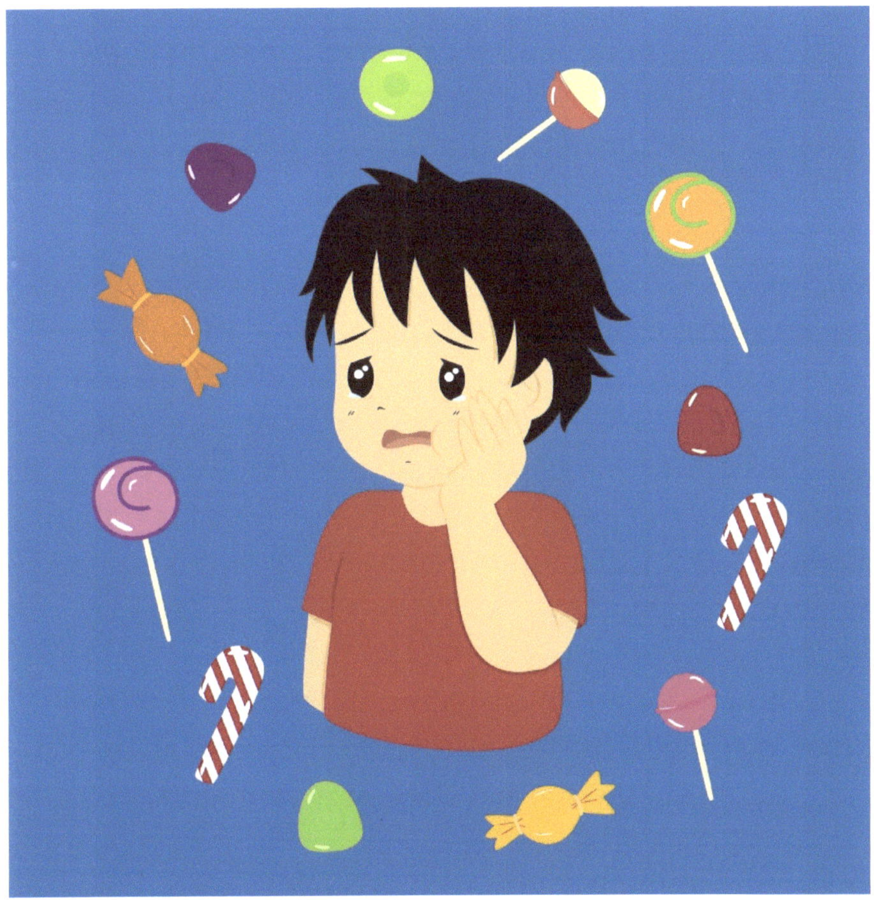

After years of denying a relation between diet and acne, and more research dermatologists are finally recognizing a small relation between some foods and acne. The strongest association is between sugar and acne. People who have more sugar in their diet, including high glycemic foods, will tend to have more acne.

The hormone route best explains the association between acne and sugars. When we eat lots of sugar or a high glycemic food, out insulin hormone spikes to manage it. It is believed that when the insulin spikes, the androgen hormones also spike or elevate. It is these darn androgen hormones that are responsible for creating more sebum (oil) on our skin.

There are also some studies that showed a relation between skim or fat-free milk and getting more acne. So it is not likely to be fat in dairy that would give acne, but maybe the lactose or glycemic load or something else. The connection between acne and dairy foods still needs further research and clarification, but for now the old adage "everything in moderation" could come into play here.

The high protein sport supplements, especially whey protein, also need further study in relation to acne, but there is some suspicion that they may worsen acne.

Drinking lots of water has always been rumored to be helpful for your skin, and while that has not been studied well by dermatologists, there seems to be no harm in trying, and it will definitely benefit some other skin issues like dry skin.

Some of my patients have been asking about the benefits of probiotics. There are early study results showing that probiotics may in fact be beneficial to our skin, whether topical or oral, but there is some debate as to how effective, and which ones or which formulation. Further studies are needed to clarify the benefits of probiotics on our skin. The theory with probiotics is that sometimes acne is worse when there is an abnormal balance of skin flora (bacteria). So, if we can correct the bacterial flora balance, then in theory, there could be less acne or other skin disease. The problem is we do not fully understand yet what constitutes a correct skin floral balance.

See Chapter 4 for information about the benefits of balancing skin pH for our skin. The relation between a good skin pH and good flora is also being studied. For now, I do recommend pH-correcting toners, which may in turn correct skin flora.

Chapter 9: More Crucial Things You Must Avoid

In Chapters 7 and 8, it was discussed that you must avoid **sun** and **sugar**, maybe **skim** and **fat-free milks**, maybe **whey protein**. So go back and read those chapters if diet or sun and their impact on acne are unclear.

Spinning Brushes:

I caution about these devices as they have very limited proof that they are helpful to our skin. I have seen in my dermatology practice, many people with acne try those brushes, regardless of the brand and get no improvement or worse acne. The concern is that the brush bristles may inflame the skin more, which can clog pores more and give more acne, or the brush bristles may retain dirt, bacteria and other microbes and just grind them deeper in our skin.

Knowing that we all have normal bacteria, yeast, and even mites living on our healthy skin, the thought of grinding them around is pretty gross. I would like to see more controlled studies employing these devices. The original purpose of these spinning brushes was to try and simulate microdermabrasion treatments for home. Microdermabrasion is a light exfoliating skin treatment done by aestheticians in spas. There is very limited data to support that microdermabrasion is effective or helpful for any skin disorders. It is certainly too gentle to correct skin scars, or most skin discolorations.

Makeup Sponges/Brushes:

Be sure and disinfect makeup sponges, brushes, or other applicators. The cold sterilization or herbicide used in hair salons, or 70% alcohol, or bleach would work. All these tools may collect dirt and microorganisms (yeast, bacteria, mites) from our skin and air between uses. If applying makeup with your hands, be sure and wash your hands prior to starting.

Certain Hormone Medications and Steroids:

While most birth control medications are helpful for acne in women, there are certain types that are not. A review of the birth control for acne research has shown that the following forms of hormonal contraception actually worsened acne in some users: Depo-Provera, Norplant, and Mirena IUD. It is also well known that ingesting (exogenous) steroids, or supplements containing steroids will likely worsen acne. Many other forms of oral contraceptives help acne.

Certain Oils, Fats and other Additives in some skin products:

Some ingredients in skin products and cosmetics should be avoided as they are considered by dermatologists to be comedogenic or acne producing.

Isopropyl isostearate – found in some bronzers
Cocoa Butter – found in moisturizers
Jojoba Oil – found in moisturizers
Myristyl Lactate – found in moisturizers
Stearic Acid – found in moisturizers
Isopropyl Myristate – found in sunscreen
Octyl Palmitate – found in sunscreen
Corn oil - found in powder makeup
Lanolin, Lanolin alcohol – found in skin creams and cleansers
Vegetable oils in vitamin E capsules

Now, what do we do with this information? I realize these chemical names are not memorable and outright boring. You could at least check your skin products and verify that they do not contain large quantities of any of these. Another important point, is just because it is not listed here, does not mean the chemical is not comedogenic or acne causing.

Unfortunately, there is limited data on this topic of what chemicals in skin products could give acne. Therefore, when a new formulation or new product becomes popular, like coconut oil and other oils recently, I would caution to test it first on small areas of the skin. In addition, trendy skin product ingredients do not always have good medical research to support that they work as well on our skin as they may in our food or for other uses.

An example of the discrepancy between heavily marketed and sold products and scientific research, would be collagen and now hyaluronic acid in creams and pills. To date, there is inadequate evidence to support that applying or ingesting collagen will benefit your skin. It is true that both collagen and hyaluronic acid may absorb water in your skin and swell it making it look more healthy or youthful, but there is no proof that they will stay in your skin as the structural support that diminishes with age.

Chapter 10: Tips For Using Prescription Acne Medications

Your doctor may prescribe you medications for your acne. For best results, you should get clear instructions on your daily routine, and know exactly what order you should take or apply your medications. Ask your doctor to write out the steps for you so it is clear. The following are quick tips for using your acne medications:

1. Write out your medication daily steps or routine
2. Keep your medications where you will remember to use them, front center bathroom counter, maybe near your hairbrush or toothbrush.
3. Avoid sun exposure when using most acne medications. Many of the antibiotics, and retinoids are sun sensitizing.
4. Take a picture of your acne medications with your smartphone, so if you have any questions about how to use them or concerns, you will be able to recall which one for your doctor.
5. Do not skip your medications. They are meant to be used daily. You will not get as good results or improve as quickly if you fail to be compliant with your regimen.
6. Report any difficulty or intolerable side effects as soon as possible to your doctor and stop the medication until the question is resolved.

7. Do not combine your prescription medications with over-the-counter or natural remedies without first checking with your doctor.
8. Do not wax or do chemical peels while using a topical or oral retinoid (Accutane, Tretinoin cream, Differin, Adapalene). You may peel too aggressively or not heal as well.
9. Be patient, sometimes it takes more than a month or two to see the full improvement on your prescription medications.
10. Use sensitive skin or mineral sunblocks and not chemical sunscreens while treating your acne or you may get irritation.

Chapter 11: How Can I Shrink My Pores?

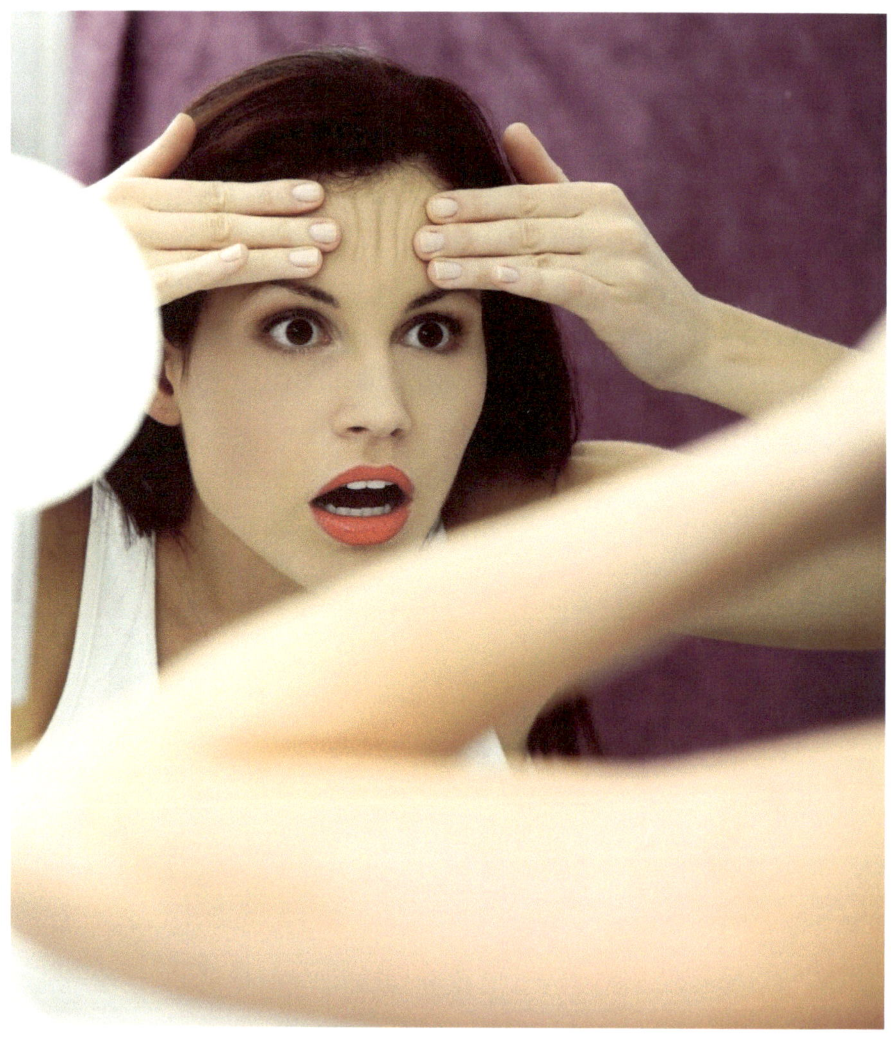

Before you get too excited, there is no surefire way to shrink one's pores, but there are ways to improve the pores. Treatments like nose strips do not literally shrink pores, but may temporarily clear them out so they are less visible. They are likely to refill 1-2 weeks later. Treatments with chemical peels also may temporarily clean out clogged pores but will not shrink the pores in any lasting way.

Topical retinoid medications used to treat acne will help reduce sebum (oil) from pores, exfoliate or shed dead skin cells from the skin which is all helpful for diminishing the size of pores during treatment, but is not permanent.

Some newer radiofrequency and laser skin treatments are suspected as capable of shrinking pores maybe even long term, but there is not enough clinical research data to prove their power yet. There is hope that within the next five to ten years these treatments will be better understood and studied and a cure for large pores will be discovered.

Chapter 12: Spa, Laser and Light Treatments for Acne

The first-line treatment for stubborn acne that does not respond to home remedies, and is more moderate or severe acne, are prescription topical and oral medications prescribed by your dermatologist. Spa, laser and light treatments are next in line and effective for most forms of acne, but they range in price from $40 to thousands of dollars.   These treatments are not usually covered by your health insurance plan, so you will have to pay upfront for them.

Often these treatments will help improve the acne faster when done in combination with the prescription treatments. In addition, spa/laser/light treatments may be used as an alternative to prescription topical and oral medications. This can be helpful where there is an allergy or intolerance to a prescription. Read on to hear more details about the laser, light and spa treatments that are typically helpful for acne.

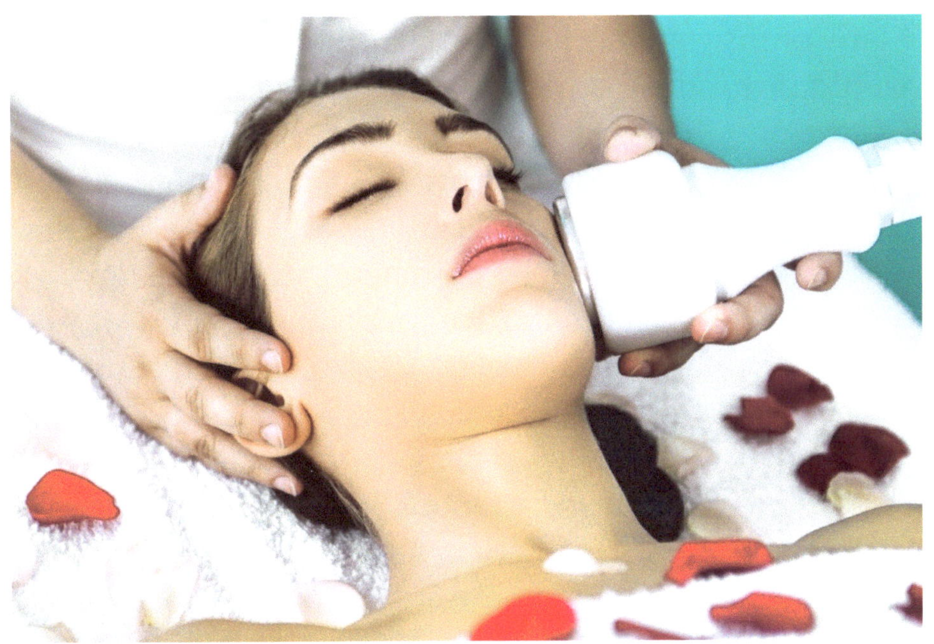

At medical spas and some medical offices, a master aesthetician can do treatments that are helpful for your acne such as chemical peels, acne extraction (pimple popping), and some gentle light and laser treatments. Chemical peels are usually meant to exfoliate the skin, which can clear out pores, fade discolorations, and smooth the skin. Unless a stronger peel done by a physician, the chemical peels effect will be mild. Gentle chemical peels may be repeated every two to four weeks for full benefit. Some physicians will offer stronger chemical peels like "Jessner's" or "TCA (Trichloroacetic acid)" which can exfoliate, fade discoloration, and smooth the skin more aggressively. This is helpful for more severe acne and acne scars.

Many of my patients ask me what the best treatment would be for their skin. There are often many good treatment options, and the choice can be very individualized and involve the following factors: skin color, medical history, medications, and your schedule. To choose the best one, I recommend you and your dermatologist discuss the pros and cons of any particular treatment for you, and guide you in choosing which treatment is best for you.

Pimple popping (acne extraction) is best done by trained hands, such as with a master aesthetician, nurse or physician. If not done properly, you may increase your risk of discoloration or scarring. If a pimple becomes infected it may fill with pus, enlarge, and be red and painful. At this time, it would be considered an abscess, and should be drained surgically by a professional. After drainage, you may be prescribed antibiotics to treat infection.

A dermatologist may also recommend injection of an inflamed pimple with an anti-inflammatory steroid medication like Kenalog (triamcinolone). Low-level light, also known as red, blue, and infrared light may improve acne. These treatments are most effective with the larger in-office lamps. There are some home light devices that offer mini alternatives to the in-office lamps and are also helpful. In general, the home mini lights require more treatments to achieve the same improvement as the larger in-office light.

Intense pulsed light (IPL) treatments (photo facials) are done in the doctor's office with either a nurse or physician. They are very helpful to calm inflamed acne, and improve discoloration.   Intense pulsed light is not as helpful for texture problems like bumpy scars. The way IPL works to improve acne is the light emitted are certain wavelengths that are absorbed by colors in the skin. Red and brown areas are inflamed with heat, which will seal a red vessel closed or peel a brown spot off. One to three treatment sessions are generally needed for best results.

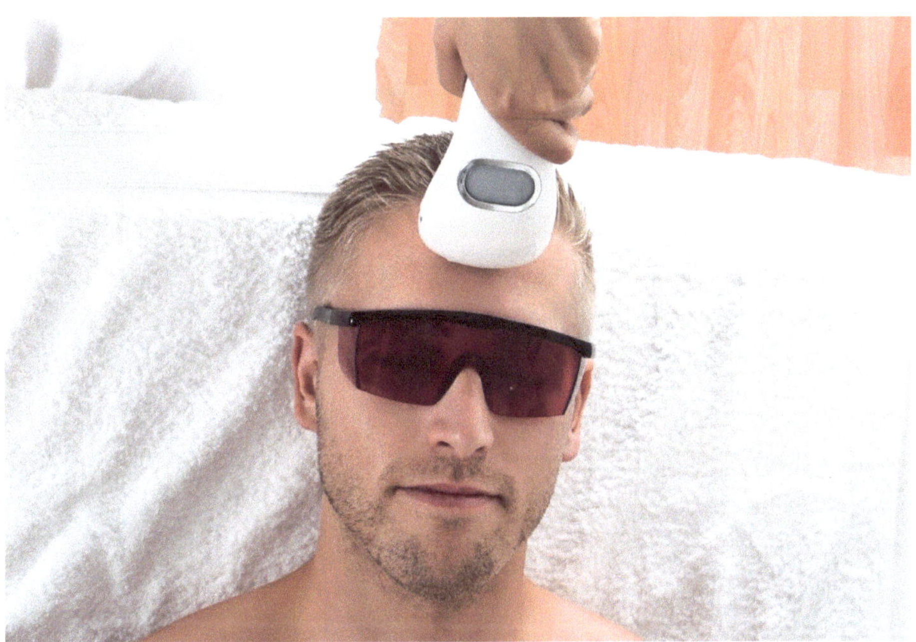

Lasers can be used to calm or improve active or inflamed acne as well as acne discoloration or scars. Some gentler laser treatments that require less healing time and repeat treatments for best results may be done by a nurse or physician assistant in a dermatology or plastic surgery practice. There are laser treatments that are more intense, produce more dramatic improvement, require more healing time but fewer repeats, and are usually performed by the physician.

Currently, the best acne scar laser treatments are often combined with a surgical treatment called subcision where the dermatologist uses a needle or needle-like tool to disrupt or cut the scar bands underneath your scarred skin. Microneedling is a different procedure, usually done by master aestheticians which can be helpful for scarring but requires many more repeat treatments to get close to the results seen with the laser and subcision treatment done by the dermatologist. All of these treatments are very safe when done by experienced professionals. See Chapter 13 for more information about managing your acne scars.

Chapter 13: Preventing and Fixing Acne Scars

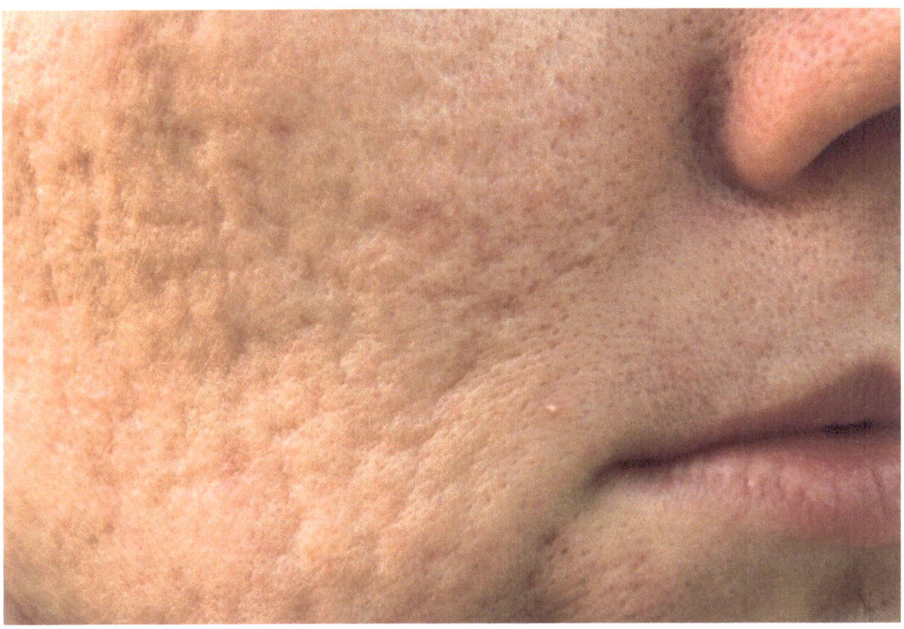

Since there is no perfect fix or cure for acne scarring, it is important to prevent acne scars with proper treatment and early identification of severe, cystic, scarring acne. If you think you have this kind of acne, you should see a dermatologist as soon as possible. Prompt treatment of severe cystic scarring acne is the past treatment. I have been saddened to see in my practice people going many years without getting help from a physician.

The most effective prescription treatment for severe, cystic, scarring acne is the oral medication called isotretinoin (formerly known as Accutane.) Except with the most severe acne, other oral treatments like antibiotics or birth control (for women) may be tried first. In some adult women, an oral medication called spironolactone is quite popular for managing acne. Acne in adult women often appears on the lower face and neck, and can result in scarring.

We do not know for sure why acne in adult women tends to occur on the lower face and neck, but there are theories among dermatologists that it is where the androgen hormone receptors are most active. In addition, the women with this acne may have excess androgen hormones, which can be tested with a blood test. Some of women also get dark hairs on our lower face and neck, which would be consistent with androgen hormone activity. This androgen hormone activity is not necessarily abnormal, but just a nuisance. Spironolactone is a blood pressure medication that has an anti-androgen hormone effect which can be very helpful for acne. Women can safely stay on spironolactone for many years, as needed, to control their acne. To learn more about spironolactone, ask your dermatologist. See Chapter 13 for laser and device treatments for severe, scarring acne.

Once you have managed or prevented your severe, cystic acne with one of the above treatments, then it is time to consider how to improve the acne scars. I usually recommend that your acne be reduced and well controlled for at least four months before considering an acne scar treatment. It does not make sense to undergo an acne scar treatment if you are still getting new scars.

Chapter 14: Natural or Home Remedies

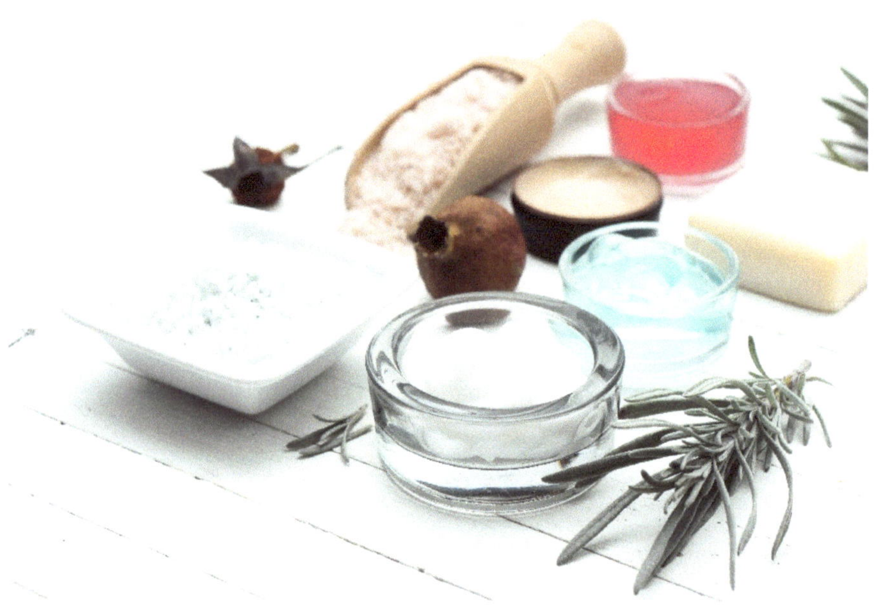

Who does not like natural and do it yourself at home? Not to mention that when you see a pimple coming on, you are usually at home and you want to do something quickly! I wish I could say that putting vinegar or bleach or toothpaste works like a charm, but none of those work very well for acne as you may have read on the internet.

Vinegar may offer some exfoliation power. Exfoliation, or shedding of dead skin cells, does help certain forms of acne, but as you know from reading the rest of this book, exfoliation plays a small role in helping most acne. In addition, using home cooking and other home products, like some essential oils, on your skin is risky as the strength and concentration may not be appropriate and safe for skin.

Essential oils are extremely popular right now. They are easy to find in many local grocery and pharmacy stores as well as on the Internet. One important caution I have for essential oils is that they may cause a skin rash known to dermatologists as "allergic or irritant contact dermatitis."

Before trying a new essential oil, I would test it on a small area of your skin for a few days to be sure you are not sensitive or allergic. The following essential oils may be helpful for acne when applied sparingly to the skin: tea tree/melaleuca, rosewood leaf, sage, lavender, lemon, and orange. Using essential oils for acne is, in my opinion, a weak remedy that does not compare to prescription acne medications that have years of research data to support their acne-fighting strength. That being said, an oil may be convenient if it is available, or may just compliment other more effective acne remedies.

Nowadays it is getting hard to distinguish what is a "natural" remedy and what is not and is man-made. Just as I cautioned with my discussion of essential oils, natural remedies may result in irritation or allergy reactions and should be tested on the skin with caution. Some acne fighting "natural ingredients" are as follows: **aloe vera, niacinamide, licorice root extract, feverfew, lemon, orange, lavender, calendula, sage, green or black tea, witch hazel, tea tree oil**. To find some current product lines that carry these ingredients, check the following online resource: www.skincreamguide.com

This concludes the Everyday Acne Care book. I truly hope that now since you have read this, you understand a lot more about acne and how to best fix it.